PALEO SECRETS
The Ultimate Beginner's Guide

By: Henrae Clark

REVEALING ALL THE SECRET BENEFITS OF THE PALEO DIET AND LIFESTYLE

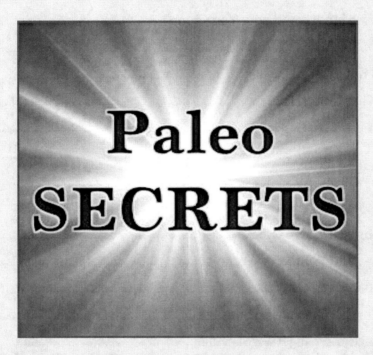

Including 50 delicious Paleo recipes and a 30 Day meal plan

Table of Contents

Introduction- The Paleo Diet

The modern industrial food we consume on a daily basis has gone through an elaborate process that is designed to make it shelf stable. While this is a commendable goal, the only problem with this approach is that only nutrients perish quickly. In other words, industrially processed food is sterile in the truest sense of the word and contains barely any nutrients, such as minerals and vitamins.

One side effect of a food without nutrients is that it also has either no flavor at all or it tastes like metal shavings. To counteract this, and make food that is actually palatable, countless millions were spent by the processed food industry to find the exact combination and quantity of chemicals that will give this kind of food the overwhelming scent, look and flavor that are supposed to mask its actual qualities.

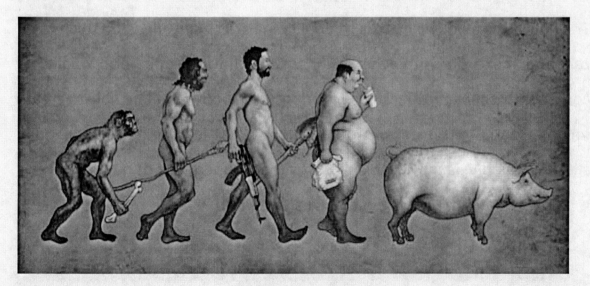

This is a highly scientific process best described by Michael Moss in his book *Salt Sugar Fat: How the Food Giants Hooked Us*. Since there is a lot of money at stake, no effort is spared in finding just the right balance of qualities to make the processed food literally addictive. For example, this includes one food giant creating a $50,000 robotic mouth used for tweaking the rigidity in potato chips so that they crunch in just the right way when eaten. Soda drinks include large quantities of sodium so that by drinking them you actually become thirstier with each mouthful. What is the end result? After finishing the current one, you yearn for another soda to quench this sudden thirst you're having.

These chemicals have an unknown effect on the human body. How does disodium phosphate affect the metabolism? What about disodium guanylate and maltodextrin? What happens when all of these chemicals are mixed together with 40 other compounds (which is the actual composition of Doritos) and consumed in large quantities daily?

The logical answer is that we literally become what we eat. Our bodies cannot create energy or the basic building blocks of the body out of nothing. The only thing a body can do is try to eliminate as many ingested toxins as it can and make do with what it has. Over time, if the food quality is consistently subpar and lacking in nutrients, the body won't be able to create most essential enzymes and other substances, leading to a total body shutdown and delayed chronic diseases that "appear out of nowhere." This is exactly what is happening in the Western world.

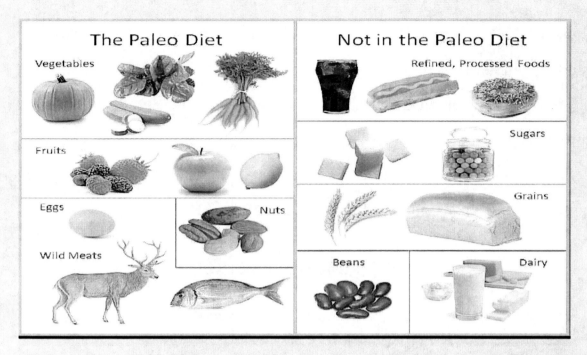

While eating corn chips and drinking soda will not kill you outright, it will cause your body's metabolism to change. At first, you will feel constantly tired and then you'll start gaining weight that simply refuses to come off. Once you fall into the rut of obesity and chronic fatigue, it becomes extremely difficult to overcome the inertia and actually make a change. To try and reverse this worrisome trend, one clever doctor suggested that we go back to the roots.

Understanding The Paleo Diet

The Paleolithic diet, also known as Paleo (pay-lee-oh), was presented in the '70s by gastroenterologist Walter L. Voegtlin and is meant to simulate the way our ancestors ate - high protein (eggs, meat, nuts) and vegetables (including fruit) without any of the "recently" introduced foods - potatoes, salt, sugar, dairy, grains and processed oils.

The reasoning behind the Paleo diet is that genes can carry habits – eating habits in particular. If our ancestors constantly ate certain kinds of foods and their diet didn't vary significantly over thousands of years, we ought to be feeding ourselves the same way for optimal health. The Paleo diet also suggests that, when we suddenly make a shift from completely natural food towards highly processed industrial food, the body enters a state of shock, which is represented by auto-immune illnesses resulting from the body almost ripping itself apart while trying to adapt.

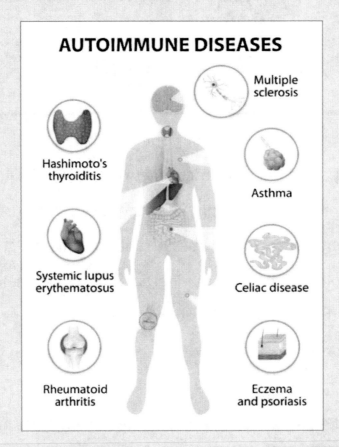

These auto-immune diseases include such horrible afflictions as lupus, rheumatoid arthritis, multiple sclerosis and vitiligo. All of these illnesses have two things in common. First, there is no treatment for them and the only thing conventional medicine can do is keep the symptoms under control and provide a somewhat normal life for the patient. Second, the common cause of all of them is a weakened intestinal lining that literally leaks food particles into the bloodstream, causing the body's immune system to go berserk and attack itself in an attempt to contain the spread.

While doctors are normally skeptical about the Paleo diet, some of them have tried it personally, out of sheer desperation, and came out of the endeavor healthy. One such story of recovery is shared by Dr. Terry Wahls in her TEDxIowaCity talk in 2011. A taekwondo champion and a mother of two, Terry was diagnosed with MS in 2000, and sought the best possible medical care.

By 2003 her disease had entered the secondary progressive phase, despite Terry undergoing chemotherapy and taking all the recommended drugs. Having no other recourse, Terry turned to reading and discovered laboratory results which showed that fish oil, creatine and Q10 halted the associated neurodegenerative processes in mice.

Terry kept researching and discovered something she had not been taught in medical school, namely the importance of proper diet to keep the body functioning well on a cellular level. This means consuming an abundance of B-complex vitamins, as well as Omega-3 oils (fish), sulfur (onions and garlic) and antioxidants. At first, she supplemented her diet with pills, but then switched over to a healthy, natural diet and eventually recovered from MS completely.

Implement the Best Paleo Solution

Habit is the strongest force known to man. When combined with hunger, it becomes an irresistible force of mythical proportions. In other words, once you get used to eating in a certain way, it is extremely difficult to change it later on, even though you might be aware that your current diet is not healthy. This is why you have to approach the matter of implementing the Paleo diet with a certain degree of meticulousness. Here is some advice for helping you to embrace the Paleo lifestyle.

Food Allowed	Food Prohibited
-Fruits	Butter
-Vegatables	-buttermilk
-Nuts	-Casein
-seeds	-Cottage Cheese
-Meat	-Custard
-Fish	-Iron Casein ate
-Etc	-Lactalbumin
	-Pasta
	-cheese
	-Oil
	-Bread
	-Grains
	-Alcohol
	-Sweets
	-Etc

Approach the Paleo diet as a way to enrich your life, rather than deprive yourself of the things you've come to enjoy and love over the years. Rather than thinking in terms "no more donuts", think, "more fruit". This will help you avoid feelings of deprivation, which lead to self-sabotage and to dropping the Paleo diet entirely.

Eating high-quality animal protein on a daily basis is a must on the Paleo diet. You should look into grass-fed organic meat suppliers and ensure you get only the best meat possible. Still, if that isn't possible on your budget, at least try to eat fresh meat regularly rather than processed food full of sugar and artificial coloring.

Fat is your friend. Though it seems counterintuitive, eating fat does not necessarily mean you will get fat. "Love handles" and "muffin tops" are caused by a rather dramatic change in metabolism caused by artificial foods and sugars, rather than plain old calorie intake. Besides, we are wired to savor fat, which means having a Paleo diet rich in coconut, avocado and lard. This will make all your meals that much more satisfying.

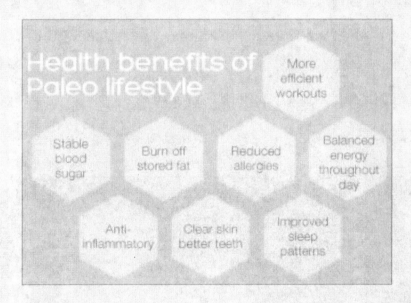

You should stay clear of Paleo baked goods. In fact, "Paleo baked" is an oxymoron, since the principles of the Paleo diet advocate eating fresh food that has known ingredients and no grain. Paleo baked muffins are at best to be considered a dessert.

Don't stress too much about setting your meal schedule. As long as you eat the food that falls within the definition of the Paleo diet, you'll be fine even if you don't eat regularly. If there is some of it left over from earlier in the day, feel free to eat it instead of a fully prepared meal.

There are other people who are going through the exact same thing as you are. Finding them and socializing with them will help you transition from the post-modern diet to Paleo. Besides, we humans consider eating a highly social event, so it will be much easier to switch from your old diet to Paleo if you do it with someone else.

Your Digestive System

If understood as a single organ, the human digestive system is the largest and most complex organ in the body, starting in the head and ending in lower abdomen. Digestion starts in the mouth, with rock-hard teeth crushing and grinding the food, which is also acted upon by enzymes found in the saliva.

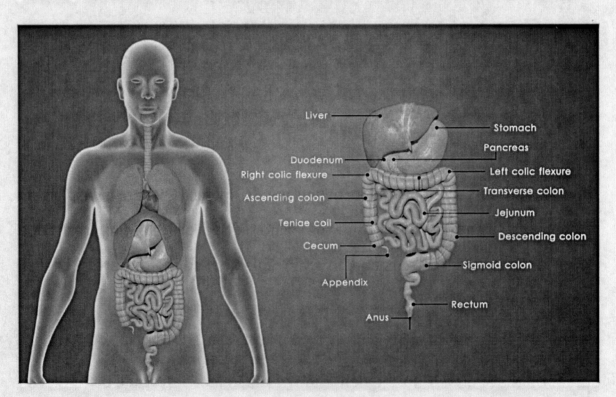

The food then travels down the esophagus with each action of swallowing. The esophagus functions in such a way that the food can't enter the windpipe, even though both openings are located right next to each other. This allows you breathe comfortably while eating.

The stomach is where the main digestion process takes place. This baggy organ is lined with cells that produce a strong acid that breaks down food and destroys harmful bacteria. The cells themselves are immune to this acid, but are usually the first thing to break down when the digestive system breaks down, causing heartburn and discomfort.

The small intestine snakes for about 7 meters (22 feet) through the abdomen and breaks down food by using a combination of slow contractions, bile from the liver, and pancreatic enzymes. This is where the food breaks down into a liquid form, and nutrients get absorbed through the intestinal wall and into the bloodstream. The residual food moves on and enters the large intestine.

The large intestine is a surprisingly efficient combination of elastic tubes that collect, solidify and dispose of all solid waste coming from the small intestine. This waste is mostly solid, and the water from it is deposited in a nearby pouch which, when suddenly emptied, pushes the contents of the colon down to the rectum.

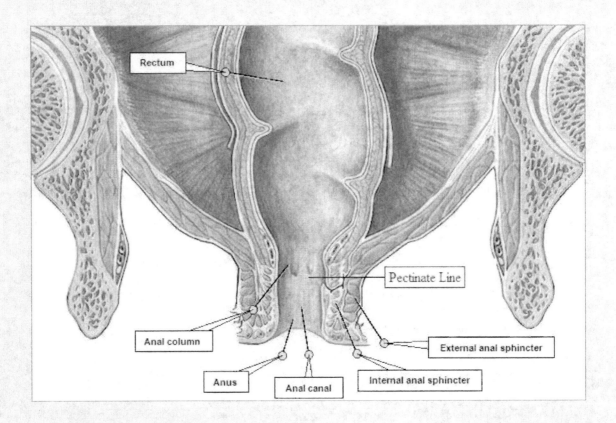

The rectum is 8 inches long and connects the colon to the anus. The walls of the rectum are particularly sensitive and will alert the relevant brain centers when anything – poop or gas – enters it. These brain centers will then decide if the pair of round muscles at the end of the anus, called sphincters, should be relaxed to let the matter through or not.

The inner sphincter is usually kept closed except when the poop arrives, and it is that which keeps us dry while we sleep, jog, read or watch cat videos on the Internet. The outer sphincter can be influenced to a degree by willpower and we can more or less decide if we want to hold the poop in or not by tightening it, though this is not recommended long term.

What do You Need to Know About Your Poop?

It is a punch line in almost all Adam Sandler comedies. It is also an extremely versatile expletive used daily in all sorts of conversations to convey shock, surprise and disgust. Yes, it's poop. There are very strong taboos around human poop – we aren't supposed to discuss it, mention it, or even look at it. There is a very good hygienic reason for that, since poop is foul smelling and foul looking due to decomposing bacteria and food remains. However, this is exactly why poop is a good indicator of health, since its purpose is to clump everything foul and unnecessary in the body in one solid piece and push it all out.

Ideally, healthy poop is brown, smooth, solid and long. If that's what you see your bowels producing, then you have nothing to worry about. Though poop travels for about a day before it gets excreted, and what you need to note is the regularity of your poop. Having a single unusual specimen is not a cause for worry, but if it's consistently unusual over several weeks or a month, you might consider visiting a doctor who will examine your intestines. Looking at your own poop and its qualities is like a free medical exam you can do in the privacy of your own home, which might literally save your life.

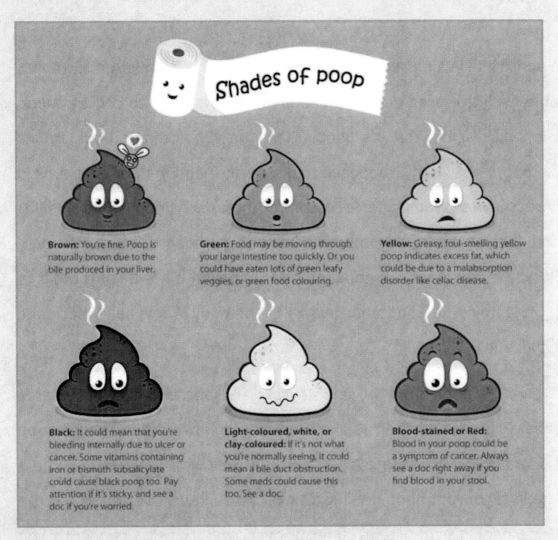

Shades of poop

Brown: You're fine. Poop is naturally brown due to the bile produced in your liver.

Green: Food may be moving through your large intestine too quickly. Or you could have eaten lots of green leafy veggies, or green food colouring.

Yellow: Greasy, foul-smelling yellow poop indicates excess fat, which could be due to a malabsorption disorder like celiac disease.

Black: It could mean that you're bleeding internally due to ulcer or cancer. Some vitamins containing iron or bismuth subsalicylate could cause black poop too. Pay attention if it's sticky, and see a doc if you're worried.

Light-coloured, white, or clay-coloured: If it's not what you're normally seeing, it could mean a bile duct obstruction. Some meds could cause this too. See a doc.

Blood-stained or Red: Blood in your poop could be a symptom of cancer. Always see a doc right away if you find blood in your stool.

Lumpy poop indicates a lack of fiber in your diet. Since fiber helps poop move through the bowels, the degree of lumpiness can show just how much fiber you need to ingest daily until you achieve a continuous piece of poop.

If your poop has hard edges and it hurts when you're emptying your bowels, then you lack fluids. Increasing your water intake will help you lubricate the colon and help your poop achieve a smooth passage. Conversely, if your poop is all liquid, you might have diarrhea, which is how the body cleans itself when there is an infection in the gut. Again, increase your water intake or you might dehydrate. Finally, poop that sticks to the sides of the toilet bowl shows that it has too much fat in it and it indicate problems with your pancreas.

One more cause for alarm is seeing blood in your poop. If that happens over an extended period of time, you should definitely schedule an exam with your doctor. By the end of 2015, around 130,000 people in the US will experience some form of colorectal cancer, including benign polyps and outgrowths. Check your poop daily and your chances are good that you'll avoid becoming a part of this statistic.

Feeling Fat?

Are you constantly trying to straighten up your back, and suck your stomach in? It does work to a degree, giving you an appearance of a slim person. But as soon as you relax, your waistline simply collapses outwards. Looking in the mirror and trying to encourage yourself simply causes you to panic even more.

Even if you cover your belly with clothes, you're constantly reminded of it whenever you make a move. Since it is so uncomfortable and disconcerting, the bulging belly of yours may even cause you to lose confidence and start abstaining from physical activity, which simply worsens the problem. Why is this happening and is there a solution?

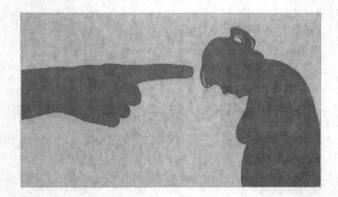

Known as "beer gut" and "love handles", this deposit of fat that happens in both men and women actually has nothing to do with drinking beer or any other kind of alcohol. Called "abdominal obesity", this phenomenon can be caused by any number of things, including hormone imbalances and lower activity levels.

Though each person should be looked at individually, the presence or absence of abdominal fat is a good indicator of overall health. Ideally, the circumference of the waist ought to be below 35 inches for women and below 40 for men. Every inch above this guideline adds to the risk of heart disease and diabetes.

The real cause of the beer belly is a surplus of calories compounded by a lack of physical activity which causes the metabolism to slow down. There is no magical solution for a beer belly save liposuction, which simply reverses the situation for a few years, but does not guarantee the beer belly won't return at a later time.

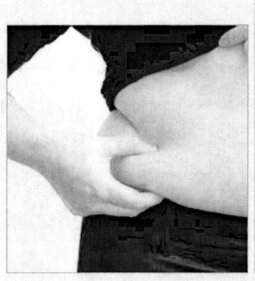

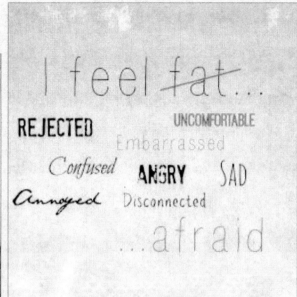

The only long-term solution for the overall feeling of "miserable fatness" caused by a beer belly is to change your diet until you're consuming small portions of high-quality natural foods, which is exactly what the Paleo diet is all about. Of course, becoming physically active won't hurt either, but you will notice actual changes once you transition away from processed food and realize that your cravings are gone forever. You will still be able to enjoy a treat or two - you just won't consider them the highlight of your day.

The good news is that the beer belly will be the first thing to go once you start doing aerobic exercise. Once you finally get rid of that massive weight around your waist, you will love lifting up your shirt and looking at the brand new slim and fabulous you.

Let's Cure the Gut

The intestines in the human body are a highly efficient organ for absorbing all the nutrients traveling through them. They possess the ability to absorb into the bloodstream only particles up to a certain size, blocking everything else. In this way, we get all the good stuff from the food we ingest. But, what happens when the intestinal wall becomes damaged?

Once the diet becomes persistently low in quality, there is a great chance that the wall of the intestines will become damaged, leading to what is known as a "leaky gut syndrome". This syndrome is exactly what its name implies, since larger particles that were never meant to enter the bloodstream can now do so.

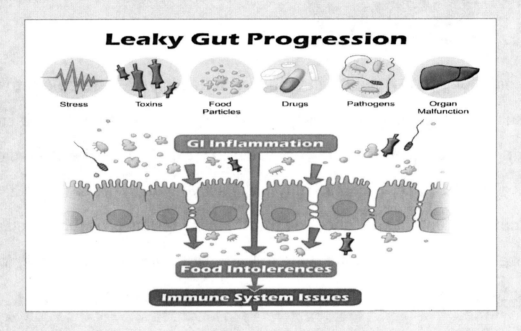

As the body's immune system detects this intrusion, it mounts a rapid response and sends out a legion of repair and protection cells that sacrifice themselves to remove these particles from the body. If the leaky gut is fixed right then and there, no permanent damage is caused and the body will eventually heal itself fully, without the person becoming aware of the problem.

However, more often than not, the leaky gut syndrome persists and begins to worsen. As more and more large particles enter the bloodstream, they start causing havoc, eventually forcing the body to attack any cells that might have come into contact with the particles. This is the beginning of an autoimmune disease.

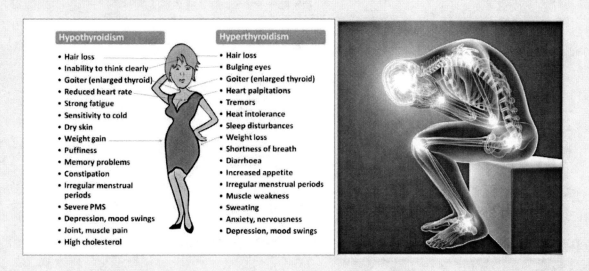

Mostly manifested as allergies, autoimmune diseases can range in severity from simply being annoying, to being debilitating and life-threatening. They can also include: sudden food sensitivities, thyroid problems leading to constant fatigue, joint pain and skin issues. For example, if you've been eating spicy food throughout your life without a problem but suddenly start getting immediate heartburn as soon as you taste chili, it might be because it's spicy food that was the first to leak through your gut and enter the bloodstream, causing the body to mount an immune response every time you eat spicy food. In any case, modern medicine ignores the "leaky gut" syndrome and aims at keeping the symptoms under control by prescribing costly medicine that does little to fix the underlying issue.

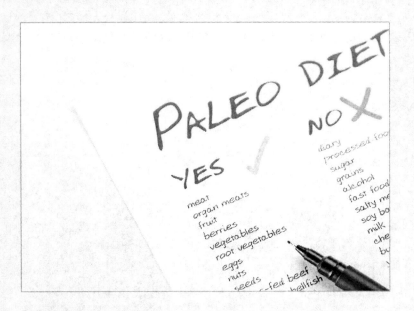

By switching to the Paleo diet, you will eliminate the majority of these particles that used to leak through your gut. Over time, your gut will recover and the symptoms will "miraculously" withdraw all by themselves. Then, you will be able to enjoy your favorite foods once again. In moderation of course.

Understand What Gluten Is

When the leaky gut syndrome was mentioned above, it was also said that there are certain large particles that enter the bloodstream and cause mayhem by finding themselves in places where they aren't supposed to be. One such particle is gluten and it caused a major fad of "gluten-free" meals, drinks, clothes, haircuts...

Though funny as it may be to cast all the blame on gluten as being the sole cause of our problems, the situation is much more nuanced. There is a number of such large particles and, though gluten is just one of them, it is the most commonly found one. Gluten is derived from grains (wheat in particular) and is found absolutely everywhere. Of course, the most abundant sources of gluten are bread, pastry and pasta. How often do you consume bread, pastry and pasta?

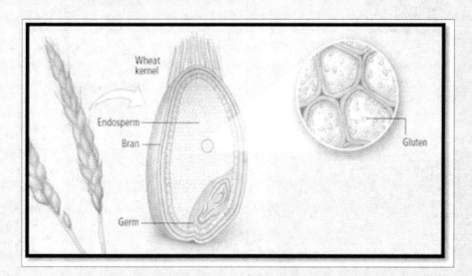

The most extreme example of gluten intolerance is celiac disease. Those stricken by it have an immense reaction when eating anything containing gluten, as their body desperately tries to prevent these particles from reaching the intestines and entering the bloodstream.

Previously thought to be genetic and unpreventable, scientists were startled when they realized that people who had been monitored over the course of 30 years developed celiac disease as they grew older, again confirming the theory that gluten intolerance is created through dietary habits. The scientists didn't dare suggest that diet might be at fault, instead placing the blame on absurdly vague "environmental factors". This study was published on the 27th September 2010 in the medical journal *Annals of Medicine*.

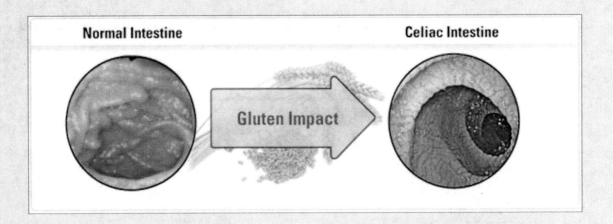

Previously unheard of, the incidence of celiac disease has doubled every 15 years since 1974 and is projected to affect 1 in 60 people in the US by 2018. But, even when it's not diagnosed as such, celiac disease strikes down many healthy persons, as it can present itself in many forms. One such form is "non-celiac gluten sensitivity", which is defined as having the same reaction that people with celiac disease have without having the same degree of intestinal damage. This again points to the fact that intestines can outwardly appear healthy while still leaking gluten particles into the bloodstream.

As always, there is another side to this story. Grains can be cultivated consistently for a relatively low cost, and provide an abundance of calories. In fact, without grains, it is doubtful that the human race would have survived its transition from being hunter-gatherers to being farmers, since the population increased while the availability of wild game decreased. Still, the Paleo diet is all about turning your life around by making a choice of diet. The bottom line is this – grains are a survival food and unless you're absolutely starving, avoid them at all costs.

Let's Go Grain Free

"Our Father (...) Give us this day our daily bread". Whether you're religious or not, you've heard this prayer and understood what it means. In simple terms, it is about humility and gratefulness for having bread to eat. While having bread definitely beats starving, the problem is that we can now grow more high-quality food than ever before and grains are a relic of the years long past.

Even better, you are now able to travel much more easily than an average person could a mere century ago, which also increases the variety of foods at your disposal. It's perfectly possible that you will eat a breakfast that comes from Japan, lunch from Paris and dinner from Canada, all the while enjoying perfectly tasty local dishes. In such a situation, why would anyone yearn for eating the same old bread that is found all around the world?

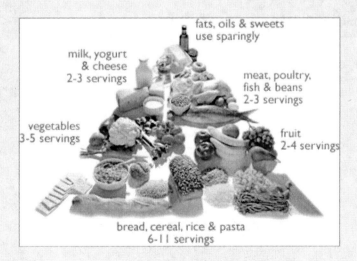

However, if you remember the elementary school curriculum, you probably were taught the "food pyramid", which had grains as the base of the pyramid. According to the "food pyramid", not only are grains good, but we can't survive without eating them daily! But that's not true at all.

While whole-grain flour might have some nutritional value that would make the damage it does to the body worthwhile, commercially purchased flour is turned into a pale shadow of whole-grain through industrial processes meant to make it shelf-stable by – you guessed it! – stripping it of all its nutrients. Ideally, harvested grain ought to be left in the field until it starts sprouting, which causes the germ to modify the chemical composition of the grain. But, since the processed food industry cares only about the biggest possible turnover, we now have flour devoid of any nutrients.

Even worse, flour causes a major blood sugar spike due to its fine structure. Though this feels great when your body releases a cocktail of hormones to deal with this sudden influx of sugars into your bloodstream, over time your endocrine glands get exhausted and cannot handle any more spikes. This in the end disturbs every single organ in the body, causing gallbladder stones and insulin resistance, among other things.

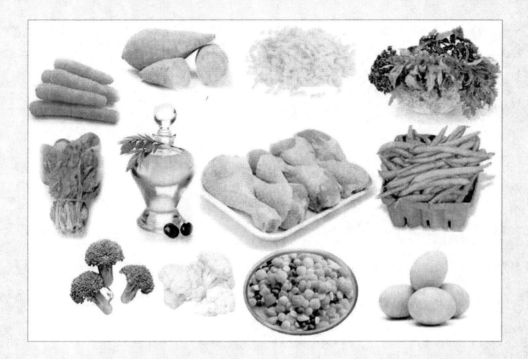

Today, modern medicine has largely moved away from cutting out the diseased organs and is more inclined to try and repair them first. But, mainstream medicine still exhibits a major mental block when it comes to actually healing the root causes of illnesses. Though it sounds cynical, it is true – medicine is a major business and having you as a repeat customer is highly lucrative. In the end, the only person who can truly care about your health is you.

Start Your Morning Right

Breakfast is the most important meal of the day. Eating a hearty breakfast lifts your spirits up and gets you ready to face all the daily challenges, whether they are in school or at work. A good Paleo breakfast could consist of a vegetable smoothie (no sugar!) and scrambled eggs cooked with lard. Naturally, you will ditch the bread or any type of dough, including pasta.

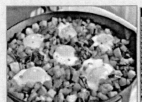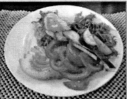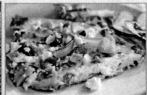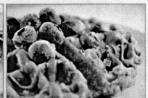

The proteins will satiate you and help your body function well, while the fats will give you a massive energy boost that does not spike blood sugar levels. Alternatively, you may opt for meat, which is available in so many forms that you never have to eat the same animal twice during a 30-day period. Fish, lamb, pork, beef and many other types of meats are completely in line with the Paleo diet. Yes, this includes bacon as well.

One more interesting thing to note is that, once you drop grains from your diet, you will start to notice the taste of the food you're eating. As a result, instead of devouring your food, you will actually start to enjoy it, making each of your meals that much more satisfying.

Adding some aerobic exercise will help you drop the extra weight, lose the beer belly and will finally give you the flexibility and zest you had as a child but gradually lost as your diet started centering on grains. Unlike all the other diets, there is no end to a Paleo diet, your Paleo meals will become a part of your life, meshed with your every choice. Rather than eating absentmindedly in front of the TV, you will savor the food and be in total control of your appetite. Having the power to simply stop after you've eaten a certain amount of food is a sensation like no other, one that will empower you and help you achieve a fuller, healthier life that you can share with your loved ones. And that's just the way it was meant to be.

In the next chapter we prepare 50 delicious Paleo recipes for you. We include all meals and many different kinds of Paleo ingredients. But, do not be afraid to experiment and to make your own unique recipes.

Ultimate Paleo Recipes

Paleo-Style Pancakes (lactose free)

If you like pancakes, crepes and hotcakes but feel too much guilt to enjoy them, here are healthy Paleo-style banana pancakes, gluten-free and lactose free.

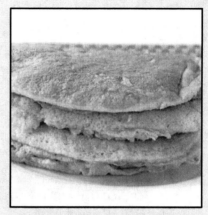

Ingredients
1 egg (large)
1 banana
1 ½ tsp almond flour
2 Tbsp. virgin coconut oil
Cinnamon

Procedure

Beat the egg. Mash the banana with a fork to reach a puree consistency and add the egg. Keep whipping. Add the cinnamon and the almond flour (ground almonds.) Pour the mixture into a small skillet greased with oil. Leave it a few seconds over high heat and then lower to the lowest setting. In a few minutes, when the batter begins to set, turn the heat back up for a couple of seconds, then lower the heat again and leave it for a couple of minutes over low heat.

If you want, you can add some fruit on top or even a bit of honey or agave syrup.

Servings: 3

Nutrition Facts

Serving size: 1/3 of a recipe (2,3 ounces).

Amount Per Serving	
Calories	145,54
Calories From Fat (69%)	99,78
	% Daily Value
Total Fat 11,53g	18%
Saturated Fat 8,47g	42%
Cholesterol 82mg	21%
Sodium 24,1mg	1%
Potassium 174,04mg	5%
Total Carbohydrates 9,41g	3%
Fiber 1,18g	5%
Sugar 4,94g	
Protein 2,82g	6%

Salted Sun-dried Tomato Crackers

Salted dried tomato crackers are simple and very tasty. Your kids will love them.

Ingredients

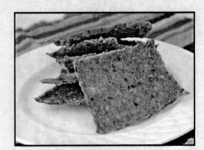

1,7 oz. sun-dried tomatoes in olive oil

1 ½ cup almond flour or ground almonds

2 oz. grated Parmesan cheese

¼ tsp salt

Oregano to taste

Procedure

Preheat oven to 280 ° F

Finely mince the dried tomatoes in the mincer. In a bowl, place the chopped tomatoes and add the almond flour, parmesan cheese and salt. Mix to form a dough. Divide the dough into 2 parts. Knead with your hands until a ball is formed. Place 1 ball on baking paper and cover with another sheet. With a rolling pin, roll out the dough to a thickness of 3mm. Remove the top sheet and cut the dough into squares the size of a cracker. Repeat with the remaining dough. Bake 20 minutes or until lightly toasted. Cool before serving.

Servings: 6

Nutrition Facts

Serving size: 1/6 of a recipe (1,4 ounces).

Amount Per Serving	
Calories	208,03
Calories From Fat (71%)	147,49
	% Daily Value
Total Fat 17,5g	27%
Saturated Fat 2,61g	13%
Cholesterol 7,33mg	2%
Sodium 240,65mg	10%
Potassium 257,97mg	7%
Total Carbohydrates 6,48g	2%
Fiber 2,98g	12%
Sugar 1,36g	
Protein 9,34g	19%

Nutty Sultana and Wolfberry Granola

There is no better way to start your day than with this extra power and vigor granola.

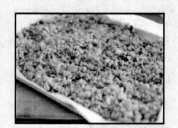

Ingredients

1 cup sultanas (or raisins)

1 cup wolfberry

½ cup almonds, slivered

½ cup walnuts, chopped

1 cup pecans, chopped

½ cup pumpkin seeds, raw

½ cup sunflower seeds

2 Tbsp. coconut oil, melted

2 Tbsp. chia seeds

2 Tbsp. flax seeds, ground

1 tsp raw honey

½ tsp cinnamon

Procedure

Preheat oven to 270° F.

In a large mixing bowl, combine sunflower seeds, pumpkin seeds, chia, flax, almonds, pecans, walnuts, coconut oil, honey and cinnamon. Stir well with a wooden spoon. Spread the blend evenly onto a baking sheet. Bake for 20 minutes.

Remove from oven and cool 10 minutes. Add in wolfberry and raisins and stir to combine.

Serve warm or room temperature with almond or coconut milk.

Servings: 10

Nutrition Facts

Serving size: 1/10 of a recipe (2,5 ounces).

Amount Per Serving	
Calories	254,92
Calories From Fat (61%)	156,5
	% Daily Value
Total Fat 18,53g	29%
Saturated Fat 4,04g	20%
Cholesterol 0mg	0%
Sodium 110,85mg	5%
Potassium 326,34mg	9%
Total Carbohydrates 21,12g	7%
Fiber 3,8g	15%
Sugar 11,74g	
Protein 5,38g	11%

Sun-up Protein Bars

Preparing these protein bars is very easy and you can put in grated coconut, chopped nuts, or chocolate chip morsels.

Ingredients

¼ Tbsp. protein powder

2 Tbsp. almond butter

1 tsp raw honey

2 tsp water

1 oz. dark chocolate chips

½ Tbsp. coconut flour

1 oz. raisins (mixed)

½ Tbsp. coconut flour

2 Tbsp. cocoa nibs

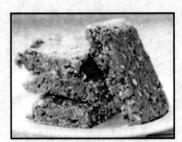

Procedure

Mix all dry ingredients in a bowl using a spatula. Set aside the water for later. After mixing well, add a teaspoon of water and keep mixing, then add another. If you find yourself needing a little more, add more until you achieve a paste consistency, without any loose ingredients being left. It is important not to pour in too much water, or the consistency will not be solid enough. Now shape the mix into small rectangles. If you see that when mixing that the dough is too sticky, then add a little more coconut flour. If it is too dry, add water. Once you have molded your bars, set them in the refrigerator for a couple of hours. You can enjoy them without having to bake!

Servings: 2

Nutrition Facts

Serving size: 1/2 of a recipe (1,7 ounces).

Amount Per Serving	
Calories	176,42
Calories From Fat (61%)	108,19
	% Daily Value
Total Fat 13,13g	20%
Saturated Fat 4,66g	23%
Cholesterol 0mg	0%
Sodium 84,71mg	4%
Potassium 205,71mg	6%
Total Carbohydrates 15,54g	5%
Fiber 3,68g	15%
Sugar 1,78g	
Protein 5,75g	12%

Sweet Potato with Greens and Sausage

This Paleo breakfast is a rich meal full of meat, eggs and veggies. It is a perfect to hold anyone over to a late dinner.

Ingredients

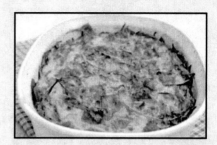

12 eggs

4 cups greens (kale, spinach)

2 sweet potatoes, diced

1 ¼ lbs. sausage

1 onion, diced

¼ cup coconut milk

½ Tbsp. coconut oil

1 tsp garlic powder

¼ tsp nutmeg

1 tsp sea salt

1 tsp pepper

Procedure

Preheat oven to 350°F. Grease a casserole dish with coconut oil.

Over medium heat, melt coconut oil and add in sausage. Stir with a wooden spoon. Set aside.

In a big bowl beat the eggs. Shred sweet potatoes and onion. Mix into eggs with seasoning, greens and coconut milk. Pour in egg mixture and stir in sausage. Cook in the oven for 40 minutes. Cover with foil and cook for 10-15 minutes more. Serve hot.

Servings: 10

Nutrition Facts

Serving size: 1/10 of a recipe (6,1 ounces).

Amount Per Serving	
Calories	166,92
Calories From Fat (41%)	69,23
	% Daily Value
Total Fat 7,77g	12%
Saturated Fat 3,17g	16%
Cholesterol 197,91mg	66%
Sodium 2722,36mg	113%
Potassium 362,24mg	10%
Total Carbohydrates 12,34g	4%
Fiber 1,32g	5%
Sugar 0,73g	
Protein 12,13g	24%

Carrot, Orange and Ginger Vigor Shake

Ginger stimulates the secretion of gastric juices and has anti-inflammatory qualities that can prevent the formation of ulcers. Also, this magic root fights skin cancer, osteoporosis, and helps weight loss. Combined, these foods also fight cellulite and help cleanse the body of toxins.

Ingredients

2 organic carrots

1 organic orange, peeled

1 piece of ginger

¼ cup of spinach (optional)

5 drops of stevia

¼ cup of ice

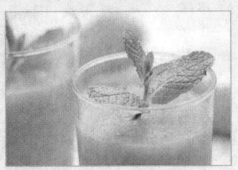

Procedure

Place all ingredients into high power blender. Blend for 2 minutes and serve.

Servings: 1

Nutrition Facts

Serving size: Entire recipe (11 ounces).

Amount Per Serving	
Calories	127,87
Calories From Fat (7%)	9,32
	% Daily Value
Total Fat 1,12g	2%
Saturated Fat 0,11g	<1%
Cholesterol 0mg	0%
Sodium 313,98mg	13%
Potassium 886,65mg	25%
Total Carbohydrates 27,8g	9%
Fiber 7,05g	28%
Sugar 15,24g	
Protein 4,65g	9%

Broiled Pine Honey Pork Chops

This elegant recipe is so versatile, and wholesome honey and garlic add a special touch to the grilled pork chops.

Ingredients

4 lean pork chops

3 cloves garlic

½ cup lemon juice

½ cup pine honey

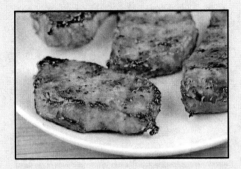

Procedure

First make a marinade. In a bowl combine all ingredients except pork chops. Put pork in a baking dish; pour marinade over pork. Refrigerate 4 hours or overnight. Before preparing the dish remove pork from marinade.

Heat remaining marinade in small saucepan over medium heat and simmer gently until the pork is ready.

Broil pork chops 12 to 15 minutes over medium heat turning once during cooking. Pour marinade over them when done. Serve hot.

Servings: 2

Nutrition Facts

Serving size: 1/2 of a recipe (11,9 ounces).

Amount Per Serving	
Calories	513,99
Calories From Fat (11%)	59,01
	% Daily Value
Total Fat 6,53g	10%
Saturated Fat 2,28g	11%
Cholesterol 122,76mg	41%
Sodium 95,91mg	4%
Potassium 844,77mg	24%
Total Carbohydrates 75,53g	25%
Fiber 0,45g	2%
Sugar 71,18g	
Protein 42,44g	85%

Coconut Lime Marinated Flank Steak

Coconut aminos is a soy-free seasoning sauce made from coconut tree sap, which comes right out of the tree so it's vital, active and alive with nutrients.

Ingredients

4 lbs. flank steak

¾ cup coconut aminos*

3 Tbsp. coconut oil

2 Tbsp. lime juice

4 garlic cloves, minced

2 tsp black pepper

1 tsp fresh ginger, grated

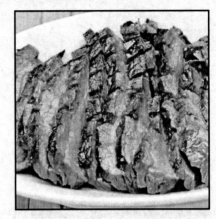

Procedure

First make the marinade: In a deep baking dish, mix all of the ingredients except the flank steak. Add the flank steak and coat in the marinade. Marinate for 10 hours in the fridge.

When the flank steak is ready, heat 1-2 tablespoon of the coconut oil in a large grill pan. Fry the steak over medium heat. Fry for 4-5 minutes per side or to preference.

Slice the steak and serve over salad.

Servings: 8

Nutrition Facts

Serving size: 1/8 of a recipe (7,4 ounces).

Amount Per Serving	
Calories	376,12
Calories From Fat (51%)	192,25
	% Daily Value
Total Fat 21,58g	33%
Saturated Fat 11,25g	56%
Cholesterol 134,95mg	45%
Sodium 107,63mg	4%
Potassium 673,41mg	19%
Total Carbohydrates 1,2g	<1%
Fiber 0,18g	<1%
Sugar 0,09g	
Protein 42,28g	85%

Garlicky Goat with Cumin and Oregano

It is almost the law that the best thing to do with goat is to marinate the meat for as long as possible, preferably overnight, and remove it from the fridge one hour before cooking.

Ingredients

4,5 lbs. goat, chopped

8 garlic cloves

2 tsp ground cumin

2 tsp sweet paprika

1 tsp ground chili

¼ cup white vinegar

¼ cup extra virgin olive oil

1 lemon, juiced

3 tsp dried oregano

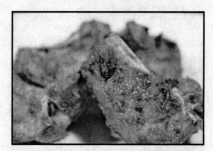

Procedure

Using a mortar and pestle beat garlic with 2 teaspoon of salt. Place in a large bowl with remaining ingredients and toss goat meat to coat in marinade. Cover with plastic wrap and leave in refrigerator preferably overnight. Remove from fridge 1 hour before cooking.

Cook goat, basting occasionally with remaining marinade, over a medium fire or coals for 45 minutes for medium or until cooked to your liking.

Servings: 6

Nutrition Facts

Serving size: 1/6 of a recipe (13,1 ounces).

Amount Per Serving	
Calories	432,69
Calories From Fat (28%)	120,69
	% Daily Value
Total Fat 13,49g	21%
Saturated Fat 3,19g	16%
Cholesterol 193,91mg	65%
Sodium 281,31mg	12%
Potassium 1367,98mg	39%
Total Carbohydrates 3,42g	1%
Fiber 0,51g	2%
Sugar 0,33g	
Protein 70,56g	141%

Grilled Lamb Chops with Spices

Make this delicious lamb chops full with herby flavors!

Ingredients

12 lamb chops

3 garlic cloves

3 tsp basil leaves

3 tsp marjoram leaves

3 tsp thyme leaves

pepper

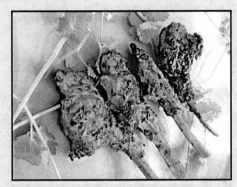

Procedure

Sprinkle lamb chops lightly with pepper. In a bowl mix herbs and mashed garlic and rub into chops. Wrap well, and chill at least 1 hour. Grill or broil 10 minutes for medium rare, 15 for medium and 20 minutes for well done.

Servings: 6

Nutrition Facts

Serving size: 1/6 of a recipe (7,5 ounces).

Amount Per Serving	
Calories	283,81
Calories From Fat (33%)	94,25
	% Daily Value
Total Fat 10,42g	16%
Saturated Fat 4,13g	21%
Cholesterol 134,4mg	45%
Sodium 135,8mg	6%
Potassium 752,89mg	22%
Total Carbohydrates 1,46g	<1%
Fiber 0,68g	3%
Sugar 0,05g	
Protein 43,26g	87%

Hot Pumpkin and Pork Stew

Stewed pumpkin and pork stew with spices and smoked paprika.

Ingredients

2,5 lb. boneless pork

3 cups pumpkin, cubed

4 dried red chilies, chopped

2 onions, sliced

4 garlic cloves, minced

1 Tbsp. coriander

2 Tbsp. smoked paprika

1 Tbsp. sea salt

1 Tbsp. oregano

½ Tbsp. black pepper

1 tsp cinnamon

3 Tbsp. fat (lard, coconut oil)

Parsley and cilantro

2oz sundried tomatoes

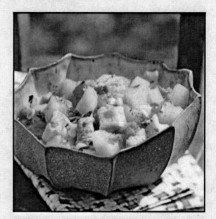

Procedure

Cut the pork into small cubes. Combine all the spices and rub the mixture onto the pork. Heat a large pot to medium high and add the cooking fat. Add the seasoned pork and cook about 7-8 minutes. Remove from the pan and set aside Add the onions, garlic, sundried tomatoes and chilies. Cook for about 2-3 minutes more. Return the pork to the pan and add about 8-10 cups of water to cover the meat. Bring to a boil, reduce heat and cook, covered, for about 3 hours.

Add the pumpkin cubes and boil gently for another 30 minutes. Garnish with roasted pumpkin seeds, chopped parsley and cilantro. Serve hot.

Servings: 10

Nutrition Facts

Serving size: 1/10 of a recipe (6,4 ounces).

Amount Per Serving	
Calories	327,78
Calories From Fat (70%)	230,1
	% Daily Value
Total Fat 25,6g	39%
Saturated Fat 8,26g	41%
Cholesterol 75,62mg	25%
Sodium 501,36mg	21%
Potassium 562,97mg	16%
Total Carbohydrates 9,61g	3%
Fiber 2,3g	9%
Sugar 2,64g	
Protein 15,68g	31%

Beef Stew with Shiitake Mushrooms and Carrots

This is a classic beef stew recipe but with silky shitake mushrooms as a delicious surprise.

Ingredients

1,5 lbs. beef meat

2 cups potato, cubed

2 cups carrot, sliced

16 oz. shiitake
mushrooms

2 cups onion, chopped

5 garlic cloves, minced

¾ tsp salt

¼ cup lemon juice

1 tsp fresh thyme,
chopped

2 Tbsp. coconut oil

2 cups water

1 bay leaf

½ tsp ground black
pepper

Fresh thyme sprigs
(optional)

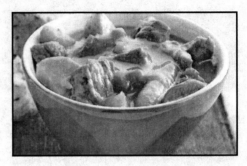

Procedure

In a large pot heat 1 teaspoon coconut oil over medium-high heat. Add shiitake mushrooms, and sauté for 5 minutes. When ready, put mushrooms into a large bowl and set aside.

In a pan, add coconut oil and onion; sauté until tender and golden brown. Add garlic; sauté 1 minute more. Add onion mixture to mushrooms

In a big pot add beef cubes with 4-5 tablespoon water; sprinkle with salt. Cook about 8-10 minutes. Mix beef with mushroom mixture. Add thyme, water, and bay leaf and bring to a boil. Reduce heat to medium-low, and simmer for 1 hour or until beef is just tender. Stir in potato and carrot. Simmer, uncovered, 1 hour and 15 minutes, stirring occasionally. Add salt and pepper to taste. Discard bay leaf. Before serving, pour in fresh lemon juice and stir well. Serve hot.

Servings: 8

Serving size: 1/8 of a recipe (10,9 ounces).

Amount Per Serving	
Calories	301,38
Calories From Fat (66%)	199,94
	% Daily Value
Total Fat 22,33g	34%
Saturated Fat 10,04g	50%
Cholesterol 48,65mg	16%
Sodium 288,11mg	12%
Potassium 461,76mg	14%
Total Carbohydrates 15,23g	5%
Fiber 2,59g	10%
Sugar 3,91g	
Protein 10,65g	21%

Boneless Lamb Hash

This hash is super-simple to pull together and loaded with spices to give you a healthy, flavorful meal in one pot.

Ingredients

2 lbs. lamb meat, cubed

4 carrots, diced

2 whole celery stalks, diced

1 onion, diced

4 cloves garlic, minced

1 can diced tomatoes

2 Tbsp. virgin coconut oil

1 cup grape juice

1 bay leaf

1 ½ tsp sea salt

1 tsp ground black pepper

1 tsp ground cinnamon

¼ tsp ground nutmeg

Fresh parsley, for topping

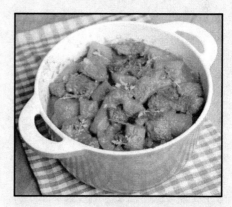

Procedure

Put the lamb in a glass bowl and season with the salt, pepper, cinnamon, and nutmeg. Place in refrigerator for up to 24 hours.

When you want to cook the lamb, using a casserole, heat the coconut oil over medium heat. Add pieces of lamb and brown on all sides. When the meat is browned, add the onion, garlic, carrots and celery. Cook for about five minutes, stirring often, until vegetables start to soften. Add the tomatoes, wine and bay leaf, and stir till mixture begins to boil. Reduce the heat to low, cover, and cook for about 2 hours. Serve hot with fresh chopped parsley.

Servings: 6

Mackerel Salad in Peppercorn Pickle

Mackerel can be prepared in different ways and in different dishes: grilled, tossed in a salad, in vinaigrette, baked, pickled...

Ingredients

2 mackerel fillets

3 Tbsp. coconut oil

3 onions, chop

2 carrots, chop

5 garlic cloves, crush

20 peppercorns

2 bunches thyme

4 bay leaves

1 cup rice vinegar

1 cup water

Salt, lettuce, arugula

1 tomato

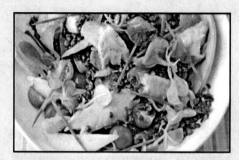

Procedure

First cook the mackerel fillets. In a frying skillet, heat 1 tablespoon coconut oil and fry the mackerel on both sides. Set aside. Fry the onions, garlic and carrots in the same skillet with a little more oil. Add the peppercorns, thyme, bay, vinegar and water. Cook for 10 min to make a pickling liquid. Cut the mackerel into coarse chunks, add mackerel to the liquid, then turn off heat. Set aside to cool. Make a salad by mixing lettuce, arugula, and tomato. Drain the fish and vegetables once cooled and add to the top of the salad.

Servings: 4

Nutrition Facts

Serving size: 1/4 of a recipe (18,6 ounces).

Amount Per Serving	
Calories	760,12
Calories From Fat (60%)	456,31
	% Daily Value
Total Fat 50,89g	78%
Saturated Fat 19,1g	96%
Cholesterol 170,1mg	57%
Sodium 229,37mg	10%
Potassium 1706,22mg	49%
Total Carbohydrates 40,94g	14%
Fiber 3,52g	14%
Sugar 6,74g	
Protein 56,11g	112%

Majorca Lobster Stew

A dish full of sea flavors goes very well with any green salad.

Ingredients

2 Tbsp. coconut oil

2 onions

4 garlic cloves

1 ripe tomato

2 lobsters

1-liter water

white pepper

salt

4 Tbsp. pine nuts

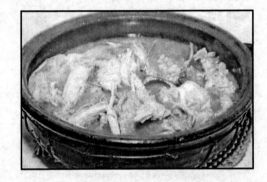

Procedure

Finely chop the onions and garlic cloves. Peel and chop the tomato. Gently fry the onions in the oil with 3 of the chopped garlic cloves, and the tomato. Cut the lobster into thick slices. Set aside the coral and roe, if any. Add the lobster flesh to the vegetable mixture, and add most of the stock. Bring to the boil and season with salt and pepper. In a mortar (or blender), crush the remaining garlic clove, the coral and roe from the lobster, and the pine nuts. Dilute with a little stock and add to the lobster and vegetables. Cook for a further 10 minutes.

Servings: 4

Nutrition Facts

Serving size: 1/4 of a recipe (23,5 ounces).

Amount Per Serving	
Calories	375,35
Calories From Fat (37%)	138,44
	% Daily Value
Total Fat 15,8g	24%
Saturated Fat 2,28g	11%
Cholesterol 290,5mg	97%
Sodium 1581,53mg	66%
Potassium 1167,59mg	33%
Total Carbohydrates 12,34g	4%
Fiber 2,56g	10%
Sugar 5,59g	
Protein 45,82g	92%

Tuna Burgers

These Paleo tuna burgers are a healthy choice for every day.

Ingredients

2 cans of tuna in oil

2 Tbsp. extra virgin olive oil

½ onion, finely chopped

2 cloves garlic, chopped

½ leek, finely chopped

½ cup tofu cheese

salt and black pepper

2 Tbsp. coconut flour

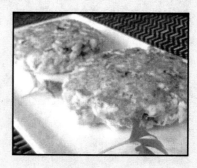

Procedure

In a frying pan, heat 1 tablespoon of the olive oil, and sauté onion, leek and garlic until translucent. Remove from the heat and set aside.

Drain tuna well. In a bowl mix tuna, onion and leek mixture, and finely chopped tofu cheese. Season with the salt and the pepper to taste.

With your hands make 4 burgers. Roll them in the coconut flour. Heat the remaining oil in a frying pan. Cook burgers over medium heat for 4 minutes on each side or until they are golden and cooked through.

Servings: 4

Nutrition Facts

Serving size: 1/4 of a recipe (3,5 ounces).

Amount Per Serving	
Calories	185.8
Calories From Fat (43%)	79,04
	% Daily Value
Total Fat 8,85g	14%
Saturated Fat 1,48g	7%
Cholesterol 11,54mg	4%
Sodium 230,31mg	10%
Potassium 189,45mg	5%
Total Carbohydrates 6,21g	2%
Fiber 0,62g	2%
Sugar 1,16g	
Protein 19,51g	39%

Salmon Fillets with Ginger-Turmeric Glaze

The lovely ginger-turmeric glaze will turn your salmon fillets into an extraordinary taste experience.

Ingredients

6 salmon fillets

4 cloves garlic, chopped

1 Tbsp. water

1 Tbsp. meadow honey

4 Tbsp. ginger, grated

2 tsp turmeric powder

Salt and pepper

1 Tbsp. fresh oregano

½ cup tomato juice

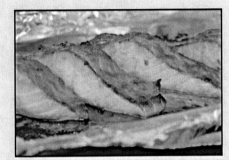

Procedure

Preheat oven to 375°F. Line a baking pan with foil and spray with cooking spray. Spray a small saucepan with cooking spray. Add the garlic and sauté over medium heat, stirring constantly, until smooth, about 3 minutes. Stir in the water, honey, ginger, turmeric, tomato juice, salt and pepper. Cook, uncovered, for 3 minutes or until slightly thickened. Arrange the salmon fillets on the baking pan. Glaze with the ginger-turmeric mixture and sprinkle with oregano. Bake for 10 to 15 minutes or until fish flakes easily with a fork. Use a spatula to move the steaks to a platter, leaving the skin on the tray. Serve hot.

Servings: 6

Nutrition Facts

Serving size: 1/6 of a recipe (4,1 ounces).

Amount Per Serving	
Calories	312,35
Calories From Fat (28%)	86,93
	% Daily Value
Total Fat 9,68g	15%
Saturated Fat 2,21g	11%
Cholesterol 129,17mg	43%
Sodium 46,07mg	2%
Potassium 900,8mg	26%
Total Carbohydrates 6,11g	2%
Fiber 0,68g	3%
Sugar 3,74g	
Protein 51,01g	102%

White Fish Ceviche with Mango

White fish in lime juice, with fresh vegetables and mango as a special ingredient. Try this combination of unique and delicious flavors.

Ingredients

2 lbs. white fish

2/3 cup lemon juice

½ cup orange juice

1 Tbsp. olive oil

1 chili pepper, chopped

1 avocado, cubed

¾ cup onions, chopped

2 mangoes, cubed

4 tomatoes, chopped

¼ cup cilantro

Salt and pepper, to taste

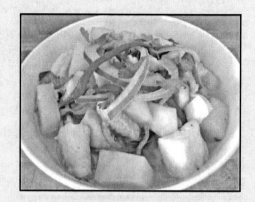

Procedure

Place fish, lemon juice, orange juice, olive oil and pepper in a glass container. Mix well, cover and refrigerate for 2 hours at least. Once the fish is marinated, add the onion and mango; set aside for 10 minutes. Remove fish from the refrigerator; add tomatoes and cilantro and season with salt and pepper.

Servings: 6

Nutrition Facts

Serving size: 1/6 of a recipe (22,2 ounces).

Amount Per Serving	
Calories	412,8
Calories From Fat (26%)	108,17
	% Daily Value
Total Fat 12,45g	19%
Saturated Fat 4,03g	20%
Cholesterol 70mg	23%
Sodium 1067,7mg	44%
Potassium 1420,55mg	41%
Total Carbohydrates 34,64g	12%
Fiber 6,73g	27%
Sugar 24,36g	
Protein 43,66g	87%

Motley Lettuce and Apple Salad

Delicious and nutritious, this is a salad full of antioxidants.

Ingredients

1 head of lettuce

4 green apples, cored

2 yellow apples, cored

1 lemon, juiced

1 stalk celery, chopped

6 radishes, sliced

½ cup pecans

50 g tofu cheese, cubed

Extra virgin olive oil

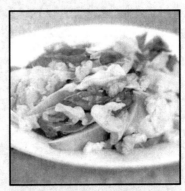

Procedure

Tear the lettuce into pieces and arrange in a bowl. Cut the apples into quarters and sprinkle with the lemon juice. Put them over the lettuce. Add the celery, radishes, cheese and pecans. Drizzle with a little olive oil. Serve immediately.

Servings: 4

Nutrition Facts

Serving size: 1/4 of a recipe (9,5 ounces).

Amount Per Serving	
Calories	263,49
Calories From Fat (41%)	108,4
	% Daily Value
Total Fat 12,91g	20%
Saturated Fat 1,81g	9%
Cholesterol 3,88mg	1%
Sodium 29,78mg	1%
Potassium 523,41mg	15%
Total Carbohydrates 37,45g	12%
Fiber 6,46g	26%
Sugar 22,96g	
Protein 5,37g	11%

Baked Carrots with Lemon

These rich and simple carrots are a perfect side dish.

Ingredients

1 ½ lb. carrots, sliced

2 onions, cut into rings

4 cloves garlic, crushed

½ lemon, juiced

1 lemon, zested

2 tsp cumin

3 Tbsp. olive oil

Ground black pepper

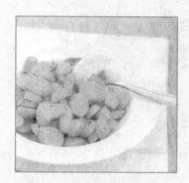

Procedure

Preheat oven to 390˚F.

Mix the carrots onion, and garlic in a bowl. In another bowl mix the lemon juice, lemon zest, cumin, oil and pepper. Pour over carrots, onions and garlic. Mix well and arrange on a tray lined with parchment paper. Bake for 25-30 minutes, occasionally stirring. Serve immediately.

Servings: 4

Nutrition Facts

Serving size: 1/4 of a recipe (3,1 ounces).

Amount Per Serving	
Calories	122
Calories From Fat (76%)	92,31
	% Daily Value
Total Fat 10,46g	16%
Saturated Fat 1,45g	7%
Cholesterol 0mg	0%
Sodium 4,91mg	<1%
Potassium 126,94mg	4%
Total Carbohydrates 7,47g	2%
Fiber 1,36g	5%
Sugar 3,07g	
Protein 0,94g	2%

Cream of Cabbage and Cauliflower Soup

This recipe is easy and quick to make. It is also delicious and full of vitamins.

Ingredients

½ white cabbage

1 leek

4 cauliflower florets

2 Tbsp. olive oil

½ tsp dried rosemary

Salt and pepper

Fresh parsley, chopped

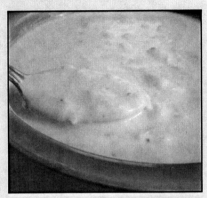

Procedure

Chop the vegetables and wash them well. Put the vegetables into a big pot and cover with water. Add olive oil, rosemary, salt and pepper, and cook for 20 minutes, until the vegetables are soft. Puree in a blender and check seasoning. Decorate with chopped parsley.

Servings: 2

Nutrition Facts

Serving size: 1/2 of a recipe (7,7 ounces).

Amount Per Serving	
Calories	186,36
Calories From Fat (66%)	122,2
	% Daily Value
Total Fat 13,84g	21%
Saturated Fat 1,94g	10%
Cholesterol 0mg	0%
Sodium 41mg	2%
Potassium 384,93mg	11%
Total Carbohydrates 15,33g	5%
Fiber 4,66g	19%
Sugar 6,5g	
Protein 2,88g	6%

Warm Spinach and Basil Salad with Walnuts

This salad is quick to make and so good for you.

Ingredients

4 cups spinach, shredded

½ cup basil, chopped

1 yellow onion, diced

2 cloves garlic, crushed

2 tomatoes, diced

¼ cup walnuts

1 Tbsp. coconut oil

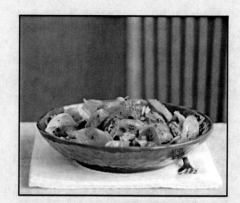

Procedure

First, wash and prepare all the vegetables.

Over medium heat, warm a small skillet. Add the coconut oil, and sauté the chopped onion until soft and translucent. Add chopped tomatoes and garlic and cook for 2-3 minutes more. Finally, add basil and the spinach and cook for two minutes.

Serve warm with walnuts over top.

Servings: 2

Nutrition Facts

Serving size: 1/2 of a recipe (9,5 ounces).

Amount Per Serving	
Calories	219
Calories From Fat (69%)	152,02
	% Daily Value
Total Fat 17,62g	27%
Saturated Fat 6,92g	35%
Cholesterol 0mg	0%
Sodium 60,5mg	3%
Potassium 805,23mg	23%
Total Carbohydrates 13,06g	4%
Fiber 4,55g	18%
Sugar 3,97g	
Protein 6,1g	12%

Roasted Red Pepper and Zucchini-Eggplant Terrine

This is the perfect dish when you want to try something new!

Ingredients

4 small eggplants

8 zucchinis

2 roasted red peppers

Olive oil

10 gelatin sheets

2 sprig fresh thyme

salt, ground black pepper

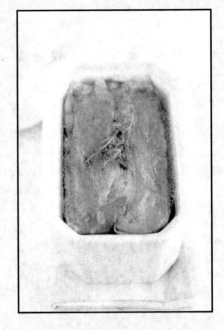

Procedure

Wash the vegetables, cut them into strips, brush with olive oil and grill them. Moisturize gelatin sheets in cold water for 10 minutes. Mix the cooking liquid from the roasted vegetables with water to make up 500ml of liquid. Put 1/3 of the liquid into a saucepan to infuse with the thyme. When hot, remove the thyme and add the drained gelatin sheets. Stir well. To assemble the terrine put strips of roasted red pepper, shredded zucchini and eggplant in rows in a terrine dish. Fill with liquid. Refrigerate for at least 24 hours. To serve, unmold and slice with a sharp hot knife.

Servings: 4

Nutrition Facts

Serving size: 1/4 of a recipe (13,6 ounces).

Amount Per Serving	
Calories	153,43
Calories From Fat (5%)	7,69
	% Daily Value
Total Fat 0,9g	1%
Saturated Fat 0,16g	<1%
Cholesterol 0mg	0%
Sodium 43,73mg	2%
Potassium 892,78mg	26%
Total Carbohydrates 21,13g	7%
Fiber 11,34g	45%
Sugar 9,5g	
Protein 19,13g	38%

Turnip Greens and Pistachio Sauté

The combination of slightly bitter turnip greens and exotic pistachios are a true taste sensation.

Ingredients

3 cups turnip greens
½ cup pistachios
1 Tbsp. coconut oil

¼ tsp salt
1/8 tsp black pepper
1 Tbsp. apple cider
    vinegar

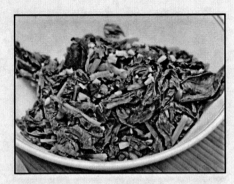

Procedure

Wash turnip greens and chop. Grind the pistachios. Heat a skillet over medium heat, and add oil when hot. Add turnip greens to the hot skillet, along with pistachios. Sauté, until the turnip leaves just begin to wilt. Stir in apple cider vinegar.

Season with sea salt and with freshly ground black pepper to taste. Serve warm.

Servings: 2

Nutrition Facts

Serving size: 1/2 of a recipe (0,4 ounces).

Amount Per Serving	
Calories	36,59
Calories From Fat (64%)	23,57
	% Daily Value
Total Fat 2,82g	4%
Saturated Fat 0,35g	2%
Cholesterol 0mg	0%
Sodium 29,38mg	1%
Potassium 70,41mg	2%
Total Carbohydrates 2,09g	<1%
Fiber 0,75g	3%
Sugar 0,5g	
Protein 1,38g	3%

All-purpose Citrus Sauce

This sauce will be the star of every dinner. Citrus juices add freshness.

Ingredients

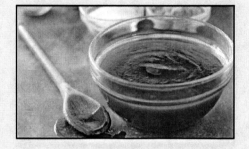

1 onion

1 tsp red chilies, finely
    chopped

¼ tsp ground red pepper

1 Tbsp. vegetable oil
    (optional)

½ cup red grapefruit
    juice

½ cup orange juice

½ cup lime juice

2 Tbsp. lemon juice

1 Tbsp. honey

1 Tbsp. cilantro,
    chopped

Procedure

In a pot heat the oil and cook onion, and red chilies, over medium heat. Cook, stirring frequently, for about 5 minutes. Stir in remaining ingredients. Bring to the boil, then reduce heat to low. Cook about 10 minutes, stirring occasionally. Enjoy over beef, pork, or chicken.

Servings: 4

Nutrition Facts

Serving size: 1/4 of a recipe (4,9 ounces).

Amount Per Serving	
Calories	94,71
Calories From Fat (34%)	32,47
	% Daily Value
Total Fat 3,68g	6%
Saturated Fat 0,29g	1%
Cholesterol 0mg	0%
Sodium 2,77mg	<1%
Potassium 204,88mg	6%
Total Carbohydrates 16,38g	5%
Fiber 0,77g	3%
Sugar 8,93g	
Protein 0,89g	2%

Cherry-Raspberry Sauce

This sweet sauce is so delicious with any kind roasted meat.

Ingredients

1/3 cup cherry juice

2 Tbsp. tapioca starch

1 cup frozen cherries
(well drained)

½ cup meadow honey

½ cup almonds

1 tsp grated orange zest

½ cup fresh raspberries

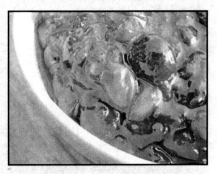

Procedure

Pour cherry juice and cornstarch into a small saucepan; mix well. Cook over medium heat until thickened. Add cherries, raspberries, honey, almonds and orange peel; mix well.

Cook over low heat, stirring frequently for about 10 minutes.

Servings: 6

Nutrition Facts

Serving size: 1/6 of a recipe (3,7 ounces).

Amount Per Serving	
Calories	226.08
Calories From Fat (24%)	54.71
	% Daily Value
Total Fat 6,54g	10%
Saturated Fat 0,63g	3%
Cholesterol 0mg	0%
Sodium 15,21mg	<1%
Potassium 152mg	4%
Total Carbohydrates 43,26g	14%
Fiber 1,42g	6%
Sugar 19,83g	
Protein 1,95g	4%

Marinara Sauce

This is a classic, tasty and very easy homemade red sauce.

Ingredients

3 cans chopped tomatoes

2 fresh tomatoes (diced)

4 Tbsp. fresh parsley

3 cloves garlic

1 tsp dried oregano

1 tsp salt

¼ tsp black pepper

6 Tbsp. olive oil

1/3 cup diced onion

½ cup white wine

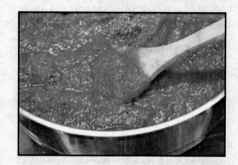

Procedure

In a blender or in a food processor, place tomatoes, chopped parsley, minced garlic, oregano, salt, and pepper. Blend until smooth.

In a frying pan sauté chopped onion in olive oil for 2 minutes over medium heat. Add the blended tomato sauce and white wine.

Cook for 30 minutes, stirring occasionally.

Servings: 8

Nutrition Facts

Serving size: 1/8 of a recipe (8,9 ounces).

Amount Per Serving	
Calories	187,39
Calories From Fat (50%)	94,26
	% Daily Value
Total Fat 10,89g	16%
Saturated Fat 1,5g	8%
Cholesterol 0mg	0%
Sodium 1012,02mg	42%
Potassium 828,86mg	24%
Total Carbohydrates 20,48g	7%
Fiber 3,77g	15%
Sugar 11,74g	
Protein 3,66g	7%

Red Pepper Sauce

This amazing sauce, whether you prefer it mild or spicy, is a delightful addition to any meal. You may add lime juice and a pinch of curry powder for added taste.

Ingredients

3 large red bell peppers

4 cloves garlic

2 Tbsp. sweet paprika

1 bunch fresh cilantro

3 Tbsp. olive oil

1 chili pepper

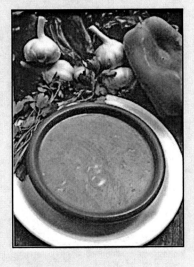

Procedure

In a high speed blender mix the bell peppers, garlic, paprika, cilantro, olive oil, chili pepper until liquefied. Refrigerate for at least one hour.

Servings: 3

Nutrition Facts

Serving size: 1/3 of a recipe (7,1 ounces).

Amount Per Serving	
Calories	138,83
Calories From Fat (61%)	84,61
	% Daily Value
Total Fat 9,57g	15%
Saturated Fat 1,3g	7%
Cholesterol 0mg	0%
Sodium 157,6mg	7%
Potassium 373,22mg	11%
Total Carbohydrates 11,88g	4%
Fiber 3,82g	15%
Sugar 6,14g	
Protein 2g	4%

Sunny Red Pepper Sauce

This bright and cheerful red pepper sauce is an excellent choice to accompany any meat or vegetables.

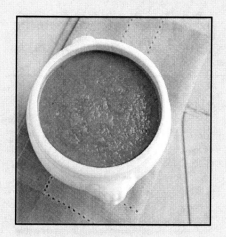

Ingredients

2 Tbsp. olive oil

1 cup chopped onion

4 large cloves garlic

1 can roasted peppers

3 anchovies, rinsed

½ cup drained tomatoes

1/3 cup ricotta

1 Tbsp. fresh parsley

Salt and ground pepper

Procedure

In a frying pan, heat the oil over medium heat. Add the onion and garlic and sauté 5 minutes, until softened. Put the onion and garlic into a blender and add the roasted peppers, anchovies, tomatoes and ricotta. Blend until smooth. Stir in the parsley and season to taste with salt and pepper.

Servings: 6

Nutrition Facts

Serving size: 1/6 of a recipe (2,5 ounces).

Amount Per Serving	
Calories	85,03
Calories From Fat (68%)	57,67
	% Daily Value
Total Fat 6,54g	10%
Saturated Fat 1,82g	9%
Cholesterol 8,67mg	3%
Sodium 115,29mg	5%
Potassium 113,34mg	3%
Total Carbohydrates 4,41g	1%
Fiber 0,72g	3%
Sugar 1,67g	
Protein 2,71g	5%

Avocado Cream with Cardamom Spiced Oranges

An extra smooth and healthy avocado cream dessert sweetened with raisins and served with spiced oranges.

Ingredients

2 avocados (fresh diced)

4 oz. pitted dried raisins

1/3 cup cocoa

Spiced orange:

2 oranges

½ cup honey

6 cardamom pods

4 cloves

2 cinnamon sticks

2Tbs. pistachios

1 Tbs. cocoa nibs

Procedure

First make the spiced oranges: Peel and segment oranges and squeeze the juice from the remaining flesh. Transfer orange pieces and juice to a small pot over medium-high heat with honey, cardamom, cloves, cinnamon and 2 tablespoons of water. Bring to the boil. Reduce heat to medium-low and cook for 15 minutes. Strain syrup through a sieve and set aside to cool. Reserve orange segments.

Second make the avocado cream: Blend the avocado, cocoa powder, raisins and reserved orange syrup in a food processor until smooth and creamy. Pour cream in four serving glasses and chill for at least 1 hour. Arrange the orange segments, pistachios and cocoa nibs on top of the cream as a garnish and serve.

Servings: 4

Nutrition Facts

Serving size: 1/4 of a recipe (9,2 ounces).

Amount Per Serving	
Calories	426,93
Calories From Fat (30%)	127,27
	% Daily Value
Total Fat 15,18g	23%
Saturated Fat 2,58g	13%
Cholesterol 0mg	0%
Sodium 18,64mg	<1%
Potassium 985,9mg	28%
Total Carbohydrates 81,53g	27%
Fiber 13,73g	55%
Sugar 58,68g	
Protein 5,36g	11%

Baked Citrus Island Bananas

This baked banana with cardamom, mashed avocado and citrus juices is an unusual but delicious dessert.

Ingredients

6 cardamom pods

3 oranges

1 lemon

6 bananas

½ cup honey

1 cup avocado

¾ cup pineapple juice

Procedure

Preheat the oven to 400°F. Remove the cardamom pods and grind the cardamom seeds in a mortar.

Squeeze oranges and lemons and put the juices in a pot along with the ground cardamom seeds, honey, mashed avocado and pineapple juice. Heat the mixture for 5-10 minutes over medium heat.

Cut bananas lengthwise and place them in a baking dish. Pour over warm juice mixture. Bake bananas for 20 minutes or until the bananas are soft. Serve at once.

Servings: 6

Cooking Time: 30 minutes

Nutrition Facts

Serving size: 1/6 of a recipe (17,7 ounces).

Amount Per Serving	
Calories	909,16
Calories From Fat (17%)	153,9
	% Daily Value
Total Fat 17,56g	27%
Saturated Fat 10,87g	54%
Cholesterol 44,79mg	15%
Sodium 10,87mg	<1%
Potassium 663,39mg	19%
Total Carbohydrates 55,55g	19%
Fiber 6,59g	26%
Sugar 37,6g	
Protein 2,74g	5%

Fruit Salad Banana Split

One of the most famous dessert sin the world can be Paleo too!

Ingredients

2 large bananas

3 cups watermelon chunks

1 pint fresh blackberries

¼ cup blueberries, chopped

¼ cup pineapple, chopped

½ cup coconut cream

¼ cup almonds, crushed

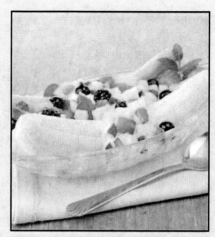

Procedure

Cut bananas in half cross wise. For each serving, lay 2 pieces of banana against the sides of a shallow dish.

Place watermelon cubes at each end of the dish. Fill center space with blackberries, pineapple and blueberries. Drizzle coconut cream over watermelon.

Sprinkle with crushed almonds.

Servings: 4

Nutrition Facts

Serving size: 1/4 of a recipe (11,6 ounces).

Amount Per Serving	
Calories	293.94
Calories From Fat (40%)	117.97
	% Daily Value
Total Fat 14,1g	22%
Saturated Fat 9,58g	48%
Cholesterol 0mg	0%
Sodium 4,19mg	<1%
Potassium 623,11mg	18%
Total Carbohydrates 44,24g	15%
Fiber 6,27g	25%
Sugar 26,86g	
Protein 4,64g	9%

Coconut Cherry Muffins

Lovely little muffins to enjoy at teatime or to take to work in your lunchbox.

Ingredients

½ cup coconut butter
    or oil

1 cup coconut sugar

1 banana, mashed

2 cups coconut flour

2 tsp baking powder

½ tsp salt

½ cup soy milk

1 tsp almond extract

2 cups cherries, pitted

1 cup almonds, toasted

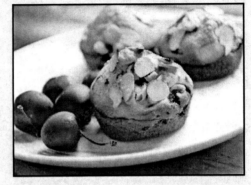

Procedure

Preheat oven to 375°F. In a big bowl blend the coconut butter and coconut sugar. Add a mashed banana and mix well.

In another bowl sift together dry ingredients and add them to the mixture. Stir almond extract into soy milk. Mix everything together, adding the almonds and cherries.

Spoon muffin batter into 12 greased muffin cups. Bake muffins for 30 minutes, or until muffins test done. Serve hot or cold.

Servings: 12

Nutrition Facts

Serving size: 1/12 of a recipe (3,4 ounces).

Amount Per Serving	
Calories	303,03
Calories From Fat (41%)	126,54
	% Daily Value
Total Fat 14,51g	22%
Saturated Fat 5,62g	28%
Cholesterol 36,65mg	12%
Sodium 190,83mg	8%
Potassium 177,99mg	5%
Total Carbohydrates 39,42g	13%
Fiber 2,3g	9%
Sugar 20,74g	
Protein 5,76g	12%

Kiwi and Strawberry Ice Pops

Paleo kiwi pops look gorgeous and they are a little bit crunchy.

Ingredients

½ cup coconut sugar

pinch of kosher salt

1 tsp cumin seeds, crushed

2 cups avocado puree

1- ½ lb. kiwi fruit, peeled

1 cup strawberries, mashed

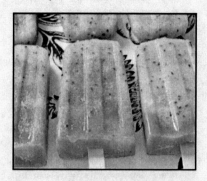

Procedure

In a saucepan over medium heat combine the coconut sugar, salt, and 1/2 cup water. Bring to a boil and add the cumin seeds. Reduce the heat and simmer for 2-3 minutes. Remove from the heat and let the syrup cool. Strain through a fine strainer into a cup, discarding the solids in the strainer. Mix avocado puree with the syrup.

In a blender, puree the kiwi and mix into the syrup/ avocado mixture. Share the strawberry mash among ten pop molds. Add the fruit and syrup mixture to each mold, filling 3/4 of the mold. Freeze until partially frozen and then insert sticks and freeze again 4 to 6 hours more.

When you want to serve, dip the mold in a deep pan of hot water until the pops pull out easily, about 1 minute. Store the pops in resealable plastic bags in a freezer and eat within 2 weeks.

Servings: 4

Nutrition Facts

Serving size: 1/4 of a recipe (8,2 ounces).

Amount Per Serving	
Calories	214,01
Calories From Fat (4%)	9,02
	% Daily Value
Total Fat 1,08g	2%
Saturated Fat 0,06g	<1%
Cholesterol 0mg	0%
Sodium 5,89mg	<1%
Potassium 595,05mg	17%
Total Carbohydrates 53,1g	18%
Fiber 6,05g	24%
Sugar 42,1g	
Protein 2,25g	5%

Sweet Rose Petal Cakes

These rose petal cakes are ideal as a dessert with a glass of chilled tea, or as a breakfast or snack.

Ingredients

3 tsp flax seed

¼ cup honey

12 rose petals, crushed

3,5 oz. coconut flour

1 tsp baking powder

½ cup applesauce

For the rose cream:

½ cup water

½ cup honey

4 rose petals

1 cup rose jam

1 tsp agar agar

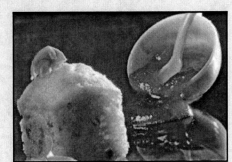

Procedure

Preheat oven to 350°F. Mix flax seeds with honey and rose petals. In another bowl mix coconut flour with the baking powder and fold into flax seeds and honey mixture. Then add the applesauce. Mix well. Pour the mixture into small cake molds. Bake for 5 to 7 minutes.

For the rose cream:

In a pot, boil the water with honey and the rose petals to make a syrup. Remove the pot from the heat and set it aside for 2-3 minutes. Add the rose jam and the agar agar. Leave to cool. Blend to a fine purée. Pour rose cream over the cakes and serve.

Servings: 8

Nutrition Facts

Serving size: 1/8 of a recipe (2,9 ounces).

Amount Per Serving	
Calories	196,4
Calories From Fat (19%)	38,26
	% Daily Value
Total Fat 4,34g	7%
Saturated Fat 0,41g	2%
Cholesterol 0mg	0%
Sodium 89,18mg	4%
Potassium 51,03mg	1%
Total Carbohydrates 40,31g	13%
Fiber 0,59g	2%
Sugar 26,05g	
Protein 1,52g	3%

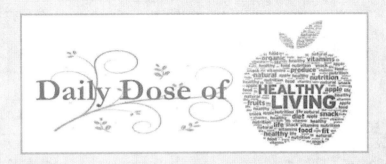

30 Day Meal Plan

Week 1			
Breakfast	**Lunch**	**Dinner**	**Snack**
Nutty Sultana and Wolfberry Granola	Garlicky Goat with Cumin and Oregano	Eggs with Walnuts and Avocado	Motley Lettuce and Apple Salad
Sun-up Protein Bars	Hot Pumpkin and Pork Stew	Tuna Burgers	Fruit Salad
Paleo-Style Pancakes	Snowy White Omelet	Easy Shrimp Stuffed Avocados	Fruit Salad Banana Split
Salted Dried Tomato Crackers	Grilled Lamb Chops with Spices	Chicken Wings with Hot Sauce	Apple and Pear Compote
Bell Pepper and Ham Omelet	Broiled Chicken with Tomato Sauce	Baked Carrots with Lemon	Turnip Greens and Pistachio Sauté
Happy Bell Pepper Omelet Muffins	Mackerel Salad in Peppercorn Pickle	Warm Spinach and Basil Salad with Walnuts	Baked Citrus Island Bananas
Vigor Carrot, Orange and Ginger Shake	White Fish Ceviche with Mango	Roasted Red Pepper and Zucchini-Eggplant Terrine	Fruit Salad
Week 2			
Breakfast	**Lunch**	**Dinner**	**Snack**
Sweet Potato with Greens and Sausage	Coconut Lime Marinated Flank Steak	Sweet Potato Gallimaufry with Fried Eggs	Kiwi and Strawberry Ice Pops
Bell Pepper Omelet	Chicken Stuffed with Hazelnut Pesto	Majorca Lobster Stew	Mixed Berry Salad

	Fried Salmon with Plum and Red Onion Salad	Chicken Skewers with Dried Figs and Rice Vinegar	Cream of Cabbage and Cauliflower Soup
Salted Dried Tomato Crackers			
Eggs with Walnuts and Avocado	Mackerel with All-purpose Citrus Sauce	Sausage with Cherry - Raspberry Sauce	Fruit Salad Banana Split
Paleo-Style Pancakes	Broiled Pine Honey Pork Chops	White Fish with Marinara Sauce	Avocado Cream with Cardamom Spiced Oranges
Salted Dried Tomato Crackers	Boneless Lamb Hash	Fried Salmon with Plum and Red Onion Salad	Turnip Greens and Pistachio Sauté
Carrot, Orange and Ginger Vigor Shake	Ground Beef Pickled Cabbage Wraps	Snowy White Omelet	Fruit Salad
Week 3			
Breakfast	**Lunch**	**Dinner**	**Snack**
Nutty Sultana and Wolfberry Granola	Ground Beef Pickled Cabbage Wraps	Bell Pepper and Ham Omelet	Warm Spinach and Basil Salad with Walnuts
White Button Mushrooms with Eggs Sauté	Boiled Beef with Red Pepper Sauce	Paleo-Style Pancakes (lactose free)	Coconut Cherry Muffins
Carrot, Orange and Ginger Vigor Shake	Boneless Lamb Hash	Chicken Wings with Hot Sauce	Mix Seasonal Fruit Salad
Happy Bell Pepper Omelet Muffins	Goose Strips with Broccoli and Cauliflower	Fried Salmon with Plum and Red Onion Salad	Baked Citrus Island Bananas
Sweet Potato with Fried Eggs	Duck Gizzards with Balsamic Vinegar	White Fish Ceviche with Mango	Apple and Pear Compote
Snowy White Omelet	Cream of Cabbage and Cauliflower Soup	Salmon Fillets with Ginger-Turmeric Glaze	Avocado Cream with Cardamom Spiced Oranges
Omelet with Sausage	Fried Salmon with Plum and Red Onion Salad	White Fish with Marinara Sauce	Turnip Greens and Pistachio Sauté
Week 4			
Breakfast	**Lunch**	**Dinner**	**Snack**
Eggs with Walnuts and Avocado	Mackerel Salad in Peppercorn Pickle	White Button Mushrooms with Eggs Sauté	Kiwi and Strawberry Ice Pops
Salted Dried Tomato Crackers	Hot Pumpkin and Pork Stew	Salmon Fillets with Ginger-Turmeric Glaze	Baked Citrus Island Bananas
Sun-up Protein Bars	Coconut Lime Marinated Flank Steak	Cream of Cabbage and Cauliflower Soup	Coconut Cherry Muffins

Paleo-Style Pancakes	Boneless Lamb Hash	Baked Carrots with Lemon	Warm Spinach and Basil Salad with Walnuts
Bell Pepper Omelet with Citrus Sauce	Broiled Chicken with Tomato Sauce	Broiled Pine Honey Pork Chops	Avocado Cream with Cardamom Spiced Orange
Carrot, Kiwi and Ginger Shake	Grilled Lamb Chops with Spices	Easy Shrimp Stuffed Avocados	Sweet Rose Petal Cakes
Nutty Sultana and Wolfberry Granola	Goose Strips with Broccoli and Cauliflower	Tuna Burgers	Mixed Fruit Salad

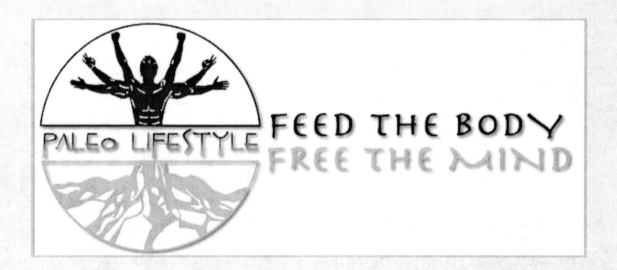

References:

http://LivingCookbook

http://paleogrubs.com/paleo-diet-food-list

http://paleoleap.com/paleo-breakfast-ideas/

http://wellnessmama.com/575/how-grains-are-killing-you-slowly/

http://mollygalbraith.com/2012/07/how-to-ease-into-a-grain-free-diet-painlessly-well-almost/

http://www.livescience.com/34990-celiac-disease-can-develop-with-aging-and-rates-are-rising.html

http://www.livescience.com/39726-what-is-gluten.html

ABOUT THE AUTHOR:

Henrae Clark is very passionate when it comes to health and dieting. With a background in physiology, nutrition, food science, and deep expertise on the benefits of paleo and gluten-free food consumption, Henrae Clark hopes to publish more books to help readers make positive changes to their lifestyle.

Henrae currently resides in Atlanta, Georgia with his wife and his puppy, Bernie. He enjoys hiking, running, traveling, and a medium-rare steak with mashed potatoes on the side.

CPSIA information can be obtained at www.ICGtesting.com
Printed in the USA
LVOW09s1452130716

496175LV00020B/423/P